HOPE

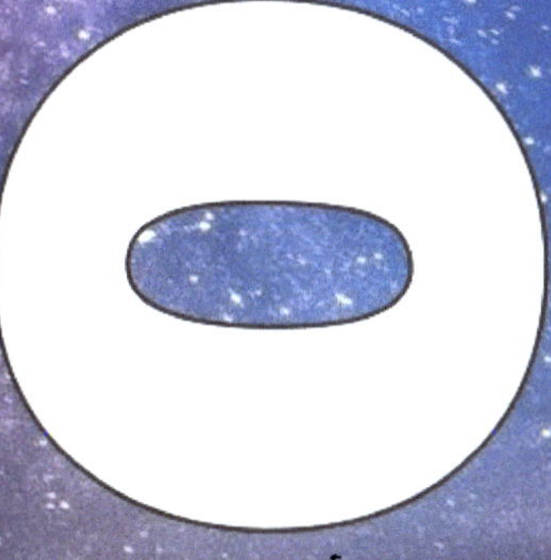

After Brain Injury

HOPE
MAGAZINE

*"Supporting the
Brain Injury Community"*

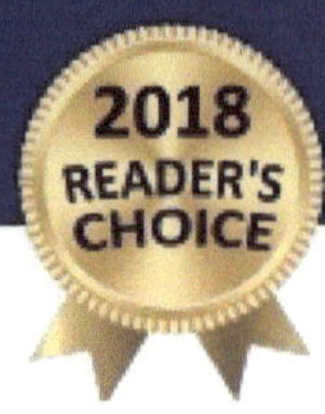

HOPE MAGAZINE

Serving the Brain Injury Community

August 2018

Publisher
David A. Grant

Editor
Sarah Grant

Contributing Writers

Haley Anderson
Nicole Bingaman
David A. Grant
Lydia Greear
Nancy Hueber
Andrew Marr
Barbara Stahura
Carole Starr
Jennifer White

FREE subscriptions at
www.HopeAfterBrainInjury.com

Welcome to the August 2018 issue of HOPE Magazine!

Over the years since we have been publishing HOPE Magazine, there have been many stories that have caused our readership to reach out to us, appreciative that a story has helped them.

In this month's issue, we are sharing a few of those inspirational stories.

Every story has value. Every story has the ability to help others. Stories are as unique as the individual – no two are alike.

It is our hope that you find something in this month's issue that helps you in your own journey. And if you are able, you can then use that experience to help someone else.

In this same light, we are always looking for survivors and those who love them, to share their stories with others through HOPE Magazine. Head over to www.HopeAfterBrainInjury.com and click on the *Submit Your Story* tab for more information.

Peace,

David A. Grant
Publisher

Contents

What's Inside

August 2018

"The greatest healing therapy is friendship and love."

~Hubert H. Humphrey

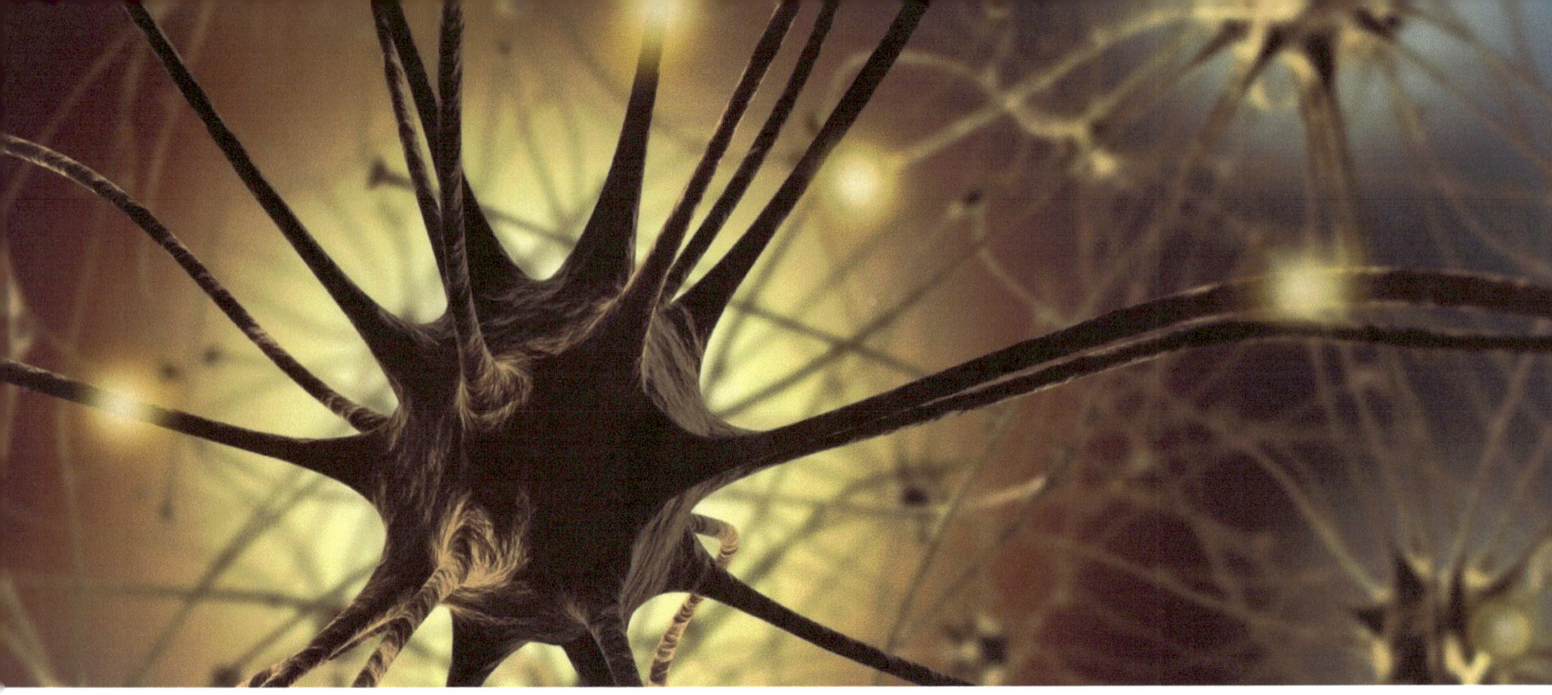

Memory

By Jennifer White

As I enter my 16th year as a survivor of a massive acquired brain injury at 36 years old, I continue to struggle to remember the things that once came easily to me. Ask me what those things are and I might say, "I cannot remember." Thankfully, most of the chilling details of my three surgeries, 10 days in ICU, a couple of weeks in the hospital and a six-month rehabilitation stay have left little memories.

Simply, I have forgotten many of the details of having the massive stroke that threw me into early retirement and changed my life forever. But, as I have lived since the ABI, I have had many memories that I will never forget, like the life and death of my mother, the day I fell down a flight of stairs as I foolishly tried to navigate the stairs while I used crutches to steady myself after breaking my femur, and the day I realized that all of the friends that I had prior to the ABI have moved on to get married, have children, become grandparents and see their children get married and have their first grandchild. I had to face the fact that I would never have children from an injury I never expected to happen to me.

> "I have forgotten many of the details of having the massive stroke that threw me into early retirement and changed my life forever."

One day I was managing my life, albeit working way too much, but going to work making everyday decisions that everyone has to make. I thought about my career, my husband, and my future. How many children would I have and when would I start having them? I also thought about social security, retirement, aging, etc. Although I still think about social security, retirement, and aging, I have, over the years, accepted my life with no children. My former friends are no longer friends who I speak with often, but memories from my past.

When I was in therapy and asked the doctors why I could not remember certain things they would tell me "you will remember the things you want to remember." They were right. I wanted to remember that I love my husband, my sister is my best friend, my brother is smart and can be really funny, and I have a good life in spite of the pain I have felt in my past.

The reality is that I had little control of my future other than trying to be a good person, doing healthy, not self-destructing things, and fighting for the things I believe in. When I was sick I had to rely on other people to help me. I let them help me, and it felt liberating to accept help from people who so unselfishly offered it.

When I struggled with memory, I designed a cardboard box and wrote the words "memory box" on the top of the box. After forgetting where I put the box almost every time I needed it, I decided that it was an idea that I should keep as an idea only. This is where I think many of my ideas should stay.

Now I practice sequencing a lot since this has been a big challenge for me. What goes first, second, etc. What time is it? For example, 8:10 AM. is earlier than 8:30 AM., but later than 7:30 AM. When I practice sequencing, it makes me feel like I am being proactive in my recovery.

"The reality is that I had little control of my future other than trying to be a good person, doing healthy, not self-destructing things, and fighting for the things I believe in."

Of course, after the ABI I felt defeated and felt sorry for myself. I constantly tried to find the answer to the question "why me?" After never getting an answer, I finally resolved the question in my head with "bad things happen to good people" and an additional question emerged. The question was "how do you want to live your life today?" I ask myself that question every morning.

Meet Jennifer White

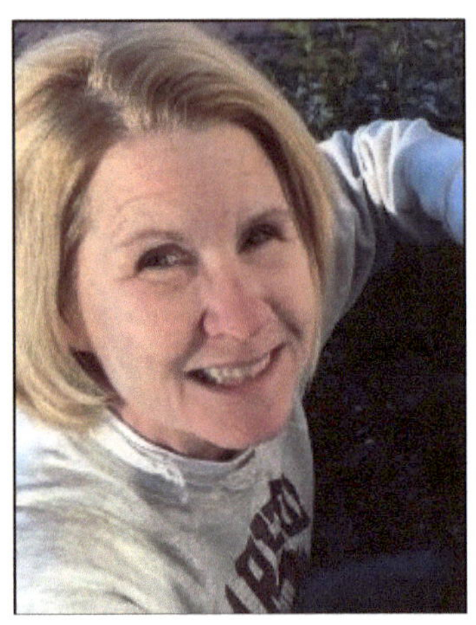

Jennifer White is an acquired brain injury survivor from St. Louis, Missouri. When she's not writing about her life as a survivor, she enjoys spending time with her family and of course, quilting.

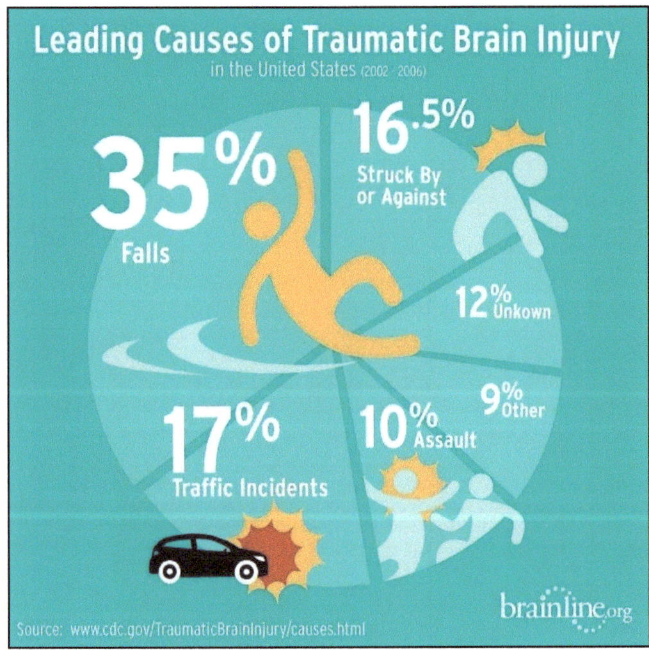

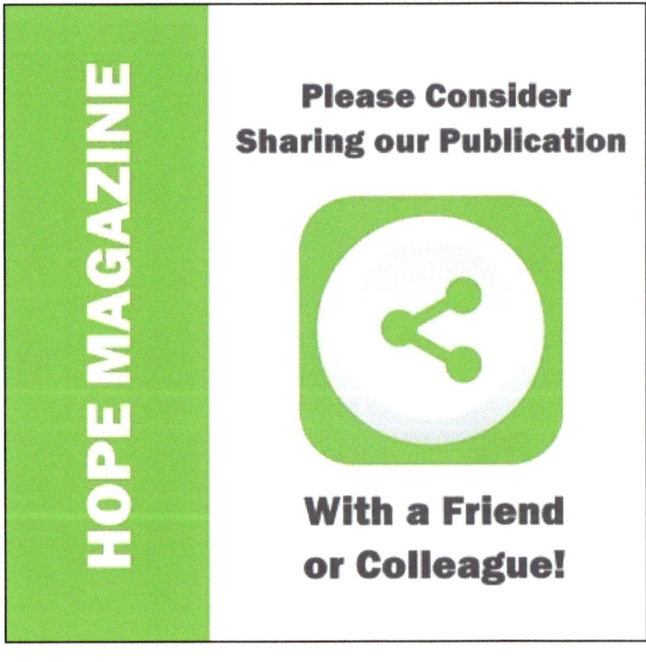

Walking with a friend in the dark is better than walking alone in the light. – Helen Keller

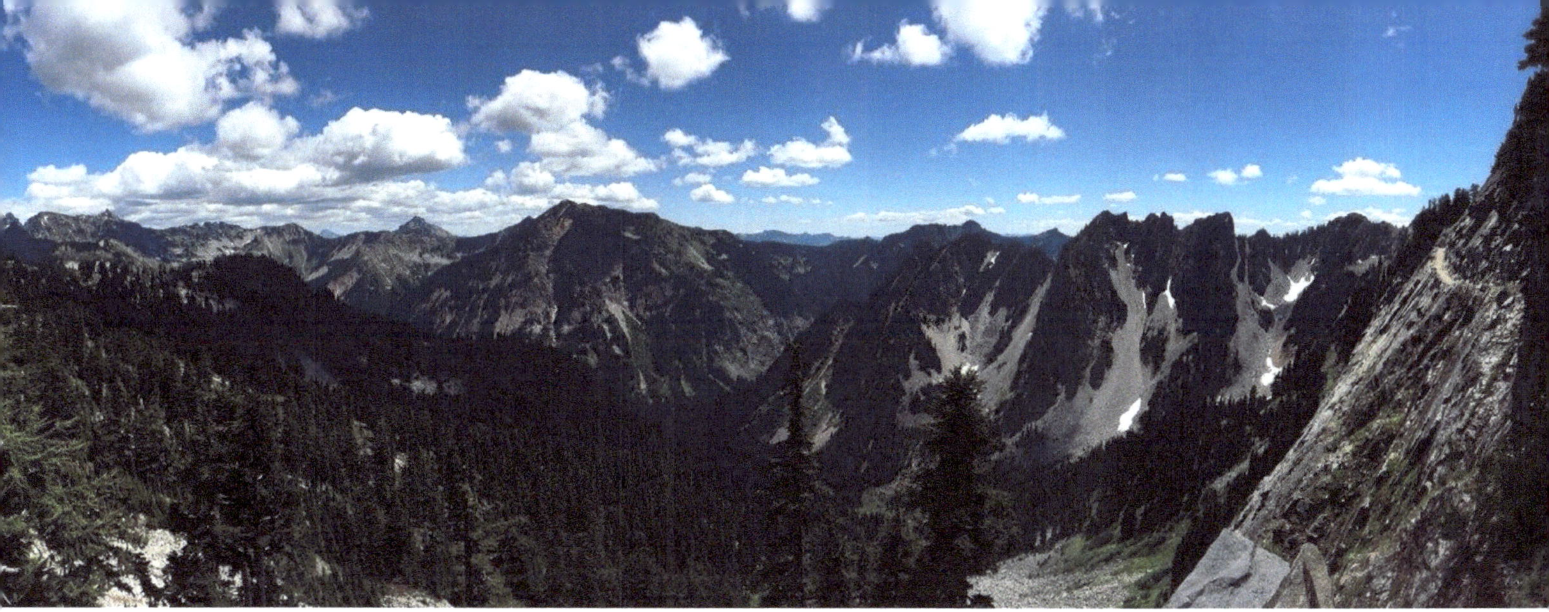

Haley's Journey

By Haley Anderson

The past two years of my life have been a rollercoaster. I sustained a Traumatic Brain Injury during my junior year of high school while on a ride in Disneyland.

After my injury, I had trouble walking and talking and had tunnel vision for nearly a year. Both my short-term and long-term memory were shot. I got intense motion sickness when I rode in the car for any longer than ten minutes and if I turned my head too fast, or even if I stood up too fast. I had a headache all day every day for months on end. I was extremely sensitive to light and sound. I put on more than 20 pounds due to various medications and inactivity. I had nightmares every night for more than a year, and I also suffered from PTSD and post-concussive syndrome. I spent the three months following my injury curled up in a ball in my room because I was in so much pain.

During the last two years I have had over two hundred medical appointments and have been treated by more than twenty medical professionals. I was not able to return to school the year of my accident.

When I attempted to return to school the following September, I wasn't sure if I would be able to graduate with my class. Fortunately, I had been an honor's student taking college classes and I was a year ahead in both math and science before my injury. Being a year ahead in my classes and taking college courses meant that I had extra credits and only needed one class - American Government - to graduate. I had an incredible teacher who would meet with me before school, after school, and during study hall to help me study and to review my notes. He was always positive and encouraging

> "I had a headache all day every day for months on end. I was extremely sensitive to light and sound."

and he believed in me when I didn't believe in myself. With his help I completed the year in baby steps and with shortened assignments. I don't know what I would have done without him.

Starting college while recovering from a head injury was a daunting task, and my parents and doctors advised me to take it slow. However, being the stubborn, high-achieving perfectionist that I am, I wanted to jump in at full speed. We all compromised and decided that I would start the quarter with two classes (a two credit *Intro to College* class and a three credit *Career and Life Planning* class). I was in denial about how bad my condition was and had convinced myself that I would be fine.

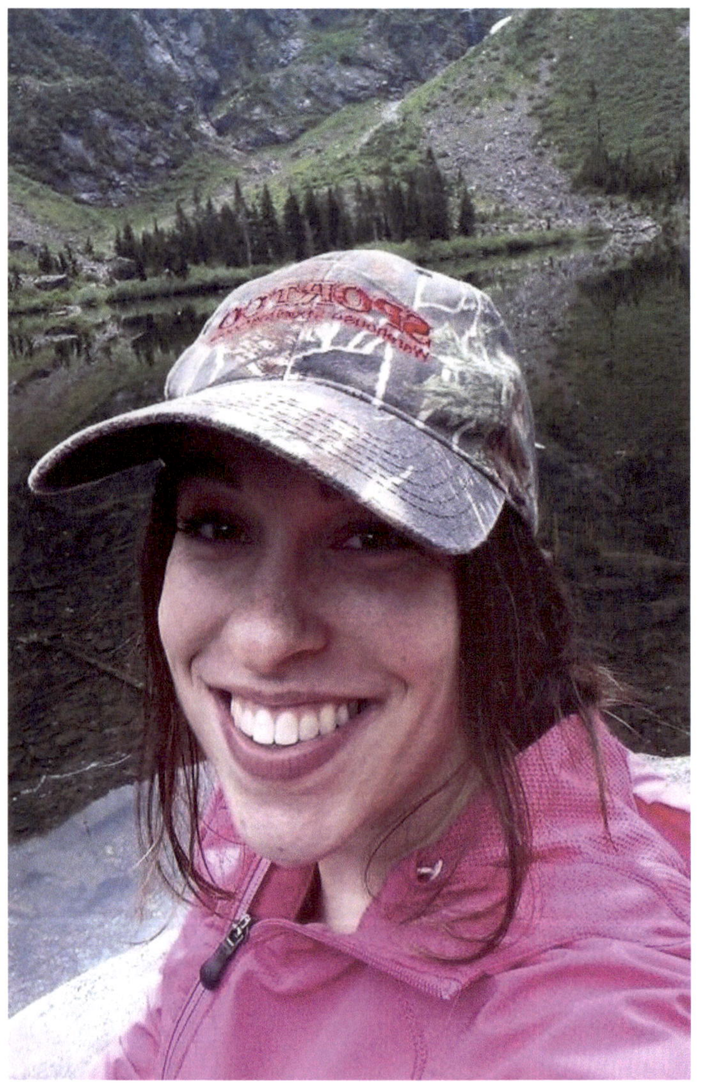

What a slap in the face the first week was. Everything that I used to do with ease (focusing in class, taking notes, keeping up with homework, remembering facts, figures, and readings from my textbook) was impossible. Despite my challenges I've managed to do well in my classes, receiving A's and B's. The thing that I struggled with the most was the realization that everything I had been able to do was dramatically altered. Working through that realization was one of the hardest things I've had to do throughout this journey and it took some time for me to adjust and to figure out how to work around my new challenges.

Working with the disability center at school has been incredibly helpful to me. I receive accommodations in the classroom (such as priority seating in the front of the class), I take my tests in a quiet room, and I also receive double time on all my tests and quizzes. My success in school this year was due to my supportive family and friends, working with the disability center, and my stubbornness and drive to succeed.

Music is my passion. In high school I played the alto saxophone, the B flat clarinet, the bass clarinet, and various percussion instruments. I was in four bands - Pep, Jazz, Wind Ensemble, and the pit orchestra for my high school's musicals. I was first chair (the highest position) and was set up to receive multiple music scholarships for college. After my injury I was forced to stop playing because playing caused intense headaches that would last for days afterwards. Recently I tried to play my alto sax for the first time in almost a year and happily realized that I could play a few notes without an immediate headache. I'm slowly increasing the time I spend playing and I'm up to five minutes now, which is so amazing and is such a big deal to me. Five minutes doesn't even begin to touch the two hours I would spend practicing in high school, but it is progress, and hey, I'll take it!

I have made great progress in the past few months. I got a job, recovered from a breakup, finished my first year at community college, found new hobbies in rock climbing and hiking, returned to rowing after a three-month break, lost the twenty pounds I had put on over the last two years. I'm down to my pre-concussion weight now, yay!

I started a new medication that helps with daily fatigue which up until recently was a HUGE problem for me. I'm also planning on picking up piano lessons again. My nightmares have subsided and I'm sleeping better at night. I've been working with a new neurologist who has been awesome and this month I'm supposed to start working with the Harborview Medical Center Neurological Rehab Program. I am so, so, SO EXCITED for that.

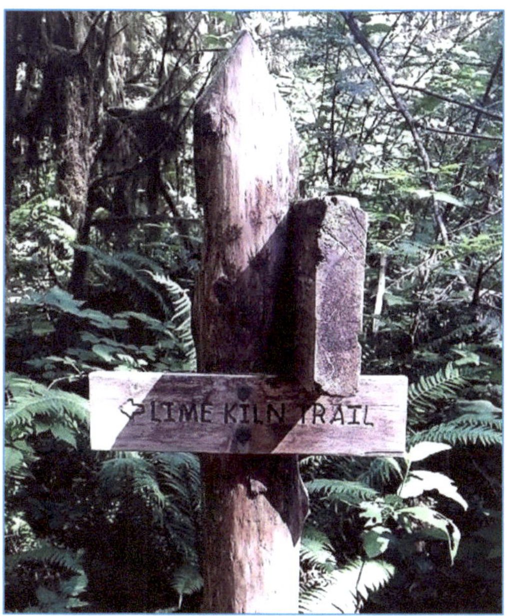

I'm naturally a happy, bubbly person and I lost that part of me after the injury. When I looked in the mirror I saw a shell of who I used to be. I looked like me, but I didn't recognize myself. Everything I held dear to me—my schooling, my music, even my relationships— had been altered and I didn't know who I was. I just felt stale and bored inside and smiling and being happy and showing emotion took so much effort that it exhausted me. As these changes have occurred I'm noticing that I'm starting to recognize the girl in the mirror again. I smile all the time and laughing is effortless. I sing in the car and laugh at bad puns and stupid jokes. The twinkle in my eyes returned. My fiery determination and happy personality came back. I feel like I can take on the world and I'm just HAPPY.

I feel really, truly optimistic for the future and what it holds for me. Right now, my plan is to finish my Associate's Degree at community college and then transfer to WSU to study Neuroscience. After I earn my degree I'd like to transfer to UW for med school to study be a Pediatric Neuropsychologist.

For the first time since my concussion I feel like ME. Others have noticed the changes within me as well. As my Dad put it, "I can see my Haley again."

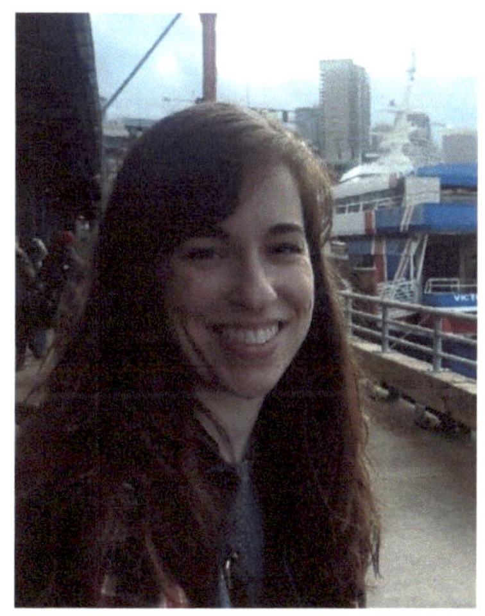

Haley Anderson is a college student currently living in Washington State and is four years post-injury. She enjoys hiking, CrossFit, painting, rowing, and camping and spending time with family and friends. Haley always has a smile on her face and her happy personality is infectious. She has faced all the challenges that life has thrown at her with grace and dignity and has not let her brain injury deter her from her goals.

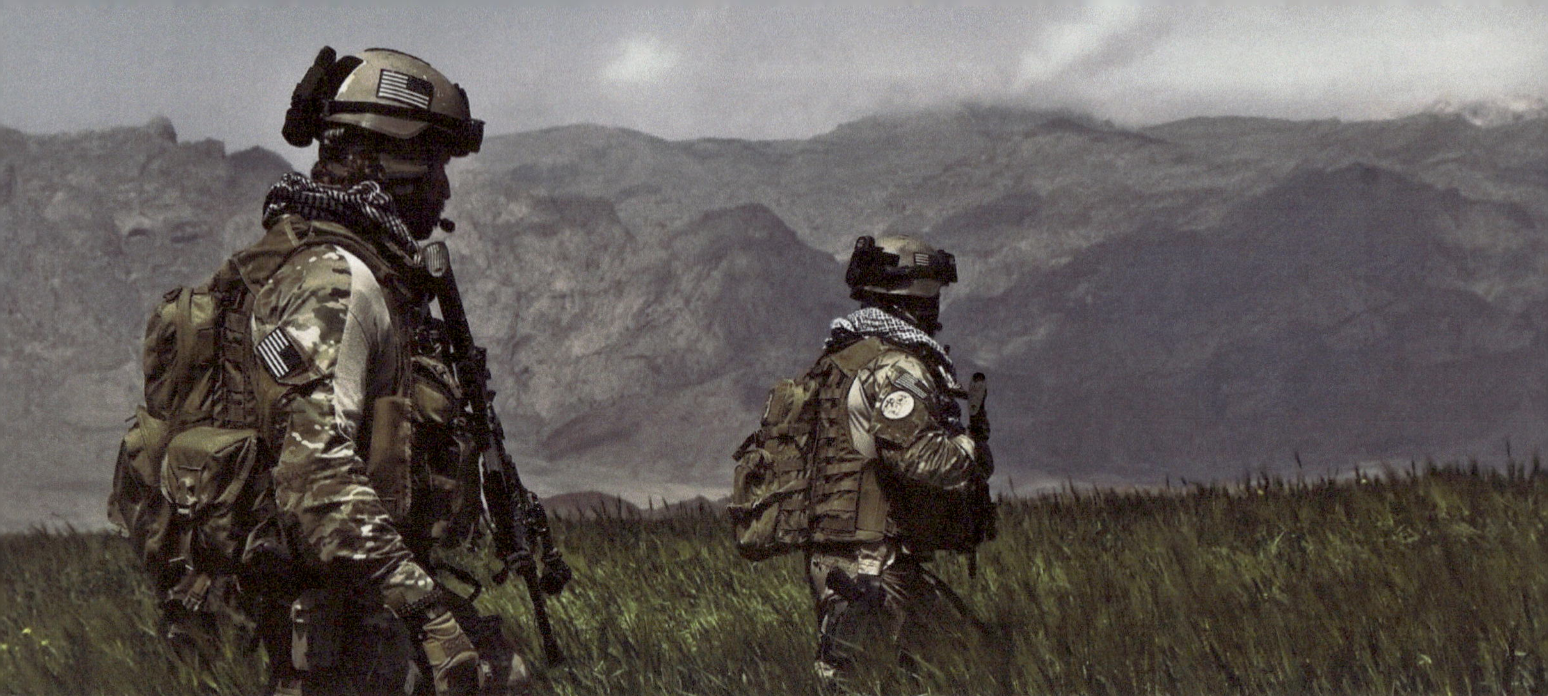

A Green Beret's Quest

By Andrew Marr

I was six months into a downward spiral and nothing was helping. After suffering numerous head traumas, I was told I could no longer take the risk of being a Special Forces Operator at the end of July, 2014. My drinking had gotten so out of control that my wife, who was nine months pregnant with our 5th child, asked me if I could keep my drinking down for the day in case she went into labor and couldn't drive herself to the hospital.

On August 31st, we had to take my thirteen-month-old son to the ER for a congenital lymphatic malformation (cyst-like formation) he had in his neck. It was infected and swollen. My wife was having contractions, and for the last three days I was dealing with what I thought was the worst calf spasm the world had ever known. All three of us were admitted into the same room in the ER.

It was ultimately decided that my son had to go to the Operating Room for surgery on his neck, and my wife went into labor not long after. My son's operation was on the fourth floor while my wife was giving birth on the second floor. I was in unbelievable pain at the time and was basically dragging my leg between the second and fourth floors to be there for both of them as much as I could. After my son's surgery, my wife gave birth. In order to be at the side of my wife and newly born son, I remember drinking and mixing opiates to combat my pain and anxiety.

> "In order to be at the side of my wife and newly born son, I remember drinking and mixing opiates to combat my pain and anxiety."

I refused treatment while my son and wife were in need. I eventually ended up in radiology to get some imaging on my calf. The imaging revealed a Deep Vein Thrombosis (big blood clot) in my leg, which by that time had broken off into a bi-lateral Pulmonary Embolism affecting both of my lungs. Had we not taken action when we did, it most certainly would have killed me. I had two hospital stays lasting several weeks, my son had over seven different hospital and ICU stays with multiple surgeries on his neck, and our newborn had a complication that required ER treatment and was admitted for four days after he stopped breathing twice. Both times my wife and I were able to revive him. All of this took place in the span of six weeks.

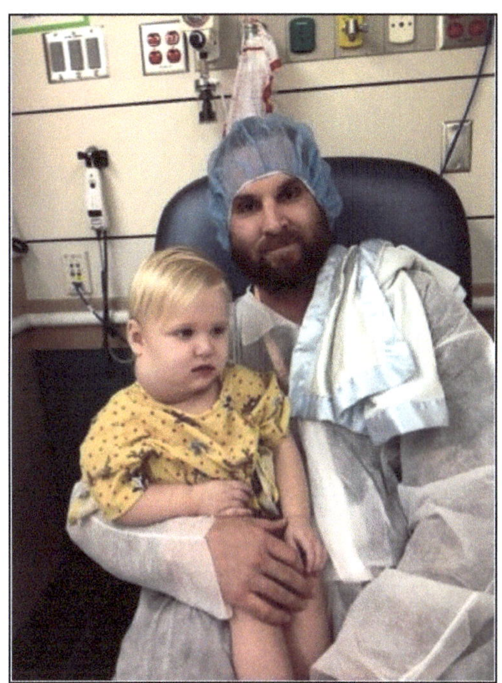

Near the midway point through that nightmare, I remember coming to a crossroads. I could blame my external circumstances and keep on the path conventional medicine had laid out for me: a path destined for my death and the destruction of my family. Or, I could embrace the current pain, accept it for what it was, and use it to improve myself. I decided to take ownership of my life and to quit allowing external obstacles to have power over me.

I then used that new-found razor-sharp focus to change what I didn't like about my current condition. From that moment on I understood that I had the power and free will to choose how I would receive, internalize, and respond to external circumstances in my life. That epiphany felt as if I had just broken free from heavy shackles, it was euphoric. I told myself that I was going to do whatever was necessary to become the man that my family and my sick boy needed me to be. I started to ask myself, "How can I make the most of every second? What must I do to improve, to be the husband, father, and leader that I require of myself?"

What Is A Traumatic Brain Injury?

We now know that the brain can suffer two distinctly different types of trauma as it relates to TBI's. The initial trauma can arrive from an external impact like an explosive blast wave, or even acceleration alone. The second and infamous "invisible injury" of a TBI occurs in the minutes and days after the initial trauma. One of the secondary injury processes that causes the biggest problem is post-traumatic inflammation.

Traumatic brain injuries can cause a host of physical, cognitive, emotional, and behavioral effects, many of which can be difficult to detect. The scientific literature tells us that symptoms can appear on impact or weeks to years following the injury.

My Last Deployment

My last deployment was in 2013. It was an emotionally and physically taxing trip. We were engaged in constant combat through the entirety of it. A majority of our team was wounded in combat before it was all said and done; my injuries resulted in a medical retirement.

My wife and I had planned on this being a relatively short trip for me. She was six months pregnant with our fourth child and first son when I left. We could not have been any happier with our life and what the future held for us. With her expected due date in early July, I planned to travel back several weeks prior to be there with her and our girls to welcome our new son into the world. It was planned that I would attend an advanced Special Forces course after the birth, keeping me stateside.

June 08, 2013

I watched an explosion blow a vehicle that weighed over 42,000 pounds, not counting our ammo or weapons, over 10 feet in the air, crashing down on its passenger side. I can still picture it in high definition and slow motion when I think about it. The very second it went off, I knew from past experiences exactly what it was. I knew the type of force that was required to send something that heavy that high into the air, and I understood the magnitude of the situation immediately.

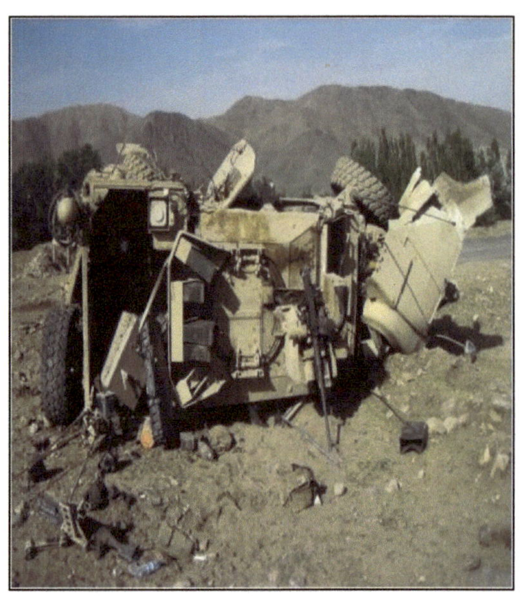

I began yelling over and over again fearing the worst. I quickly regained my composure, understanding that the probability for a follow-on attack was high. We got our ground force commander the quick update, "Let higher know that we have sustained a catastrophic IED strike on one of our vehicles, casualty report to come, we need serious air support now."

The wounds to our men, my brothers, were serious and the follow-on attack was fierce. We did what we had to do in order to hunker down and get our wounded out to the next highest level of care. It was a long day into a long night of constant combat before we finally got out of there. We didn't have the time to properly assess the number of enemy killed, but it was substantial. We made sure the enemy had every opportunity to make their ultimate sacrifice, and many did.

When we sustain a casualty, it is known that no one is to communicate with the outside world until the family members of the deceased or wounded have been notified. So once we got the go ahead that it was OK to call back home, I made the dreaded phone call.

I told my wife, "I don't know how to say this but…." and explained to her what had happened. I gave her an update on our guys. I told her that I would not be coming home, and that I would not be there for the birth of our first son. I told her that she and the kids were in a safe place and were well cared for. The guys out here were not, and I felt compelled to remain with them and continue to pursue and kill the enemy. Our survival was dependent on it. I could never face my son as a man who left his team when they needed me the most. That goes against everything I stand for, and I know one day this decision will make him proud. Becky was a seasoned veteran wife of multiple deployments, and without missing a beat she said, "I love you baby, and I am so proud of you. Do whatever you have to do, but you bring the rest of those boys back home alive. We will all be here waiting for you when you get back."

For the first time in my career, I began to video the team and me in combat on that last trip. We were walking the razor's edge out there and I knew it. I wasn't positive I was going to make it home. I wanted my boy to be able to see his Dad in action. I wanted him to have something to be proud of, something that he could actually see to let him know who his Dad was and what he was about. It was an emotionally and physically taxing trip.

The Come Down

It was about three months after my return home before I started to notice any changes. I began to be plagued by psychological, physiological, and physical manifestations, including depression, outbursts of anger, anxiety, mood swings, memory loss, inability to concentrate, learning disabilities, sleep deprivation, loss of libido, loss of lean body mass, muscular weakness, and a number of other medically documented conditions, that prior to my return had never been present.

By the time I finally came to my breaking point, I was drinking a 750ml bottle of bourbon a night, was on over a dozen medications, and had become completely detached and isolated from everyone that I loved. I was sleeping with a handle of whiskey and a loaded shotgun by my bed, dementia was quickly setting in.

The Truth

The quality of your questions can determine the quality of your life. Individual assessments using evidence-based diagnostics are required to pinpoint and treat impairments. When those methods were used on me, it changed everything. The proper diagnostic exams revealed that I had major vestibular and neuroendocrine (hormonal) deficiencies from blast-induced TBI's; however, by pinpointing the impairments we were able to effectively treat the problem. Everything up to this point had just been a Band-Aid, a temporary fix that attempted to only treat symptoms, not the root issue. We were able to get to the truth by asking quality questions. Through my treatments at Carrick Brain Centers and the Millennium TBI network I have been sober since October of last year and have come off a dozen different medications. I am performing as good if not better than my pre-injury self. My mind is clear, my body is balanced, and my spirit is grateful.

Meet Andrew Marr

Andrew is a former Special Forces Green Beret, and founder of Warrior Angels Foundation, an organization whose sole purpose is to stop the deaths of veterans suffering from PTSD symptoms caused by traumatic brain injuries. He joins us today to share that solution with you in the hopes that we can slow if not altogether stop the twenty-two veterans a day who are committing suicide thinking there is no hope or help for them. There is hope, and there is help.

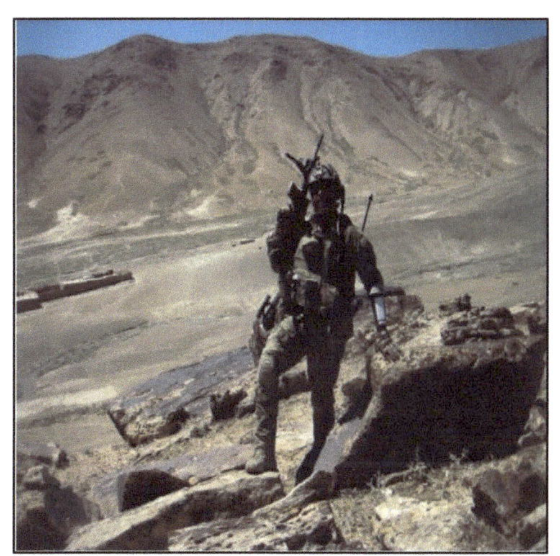

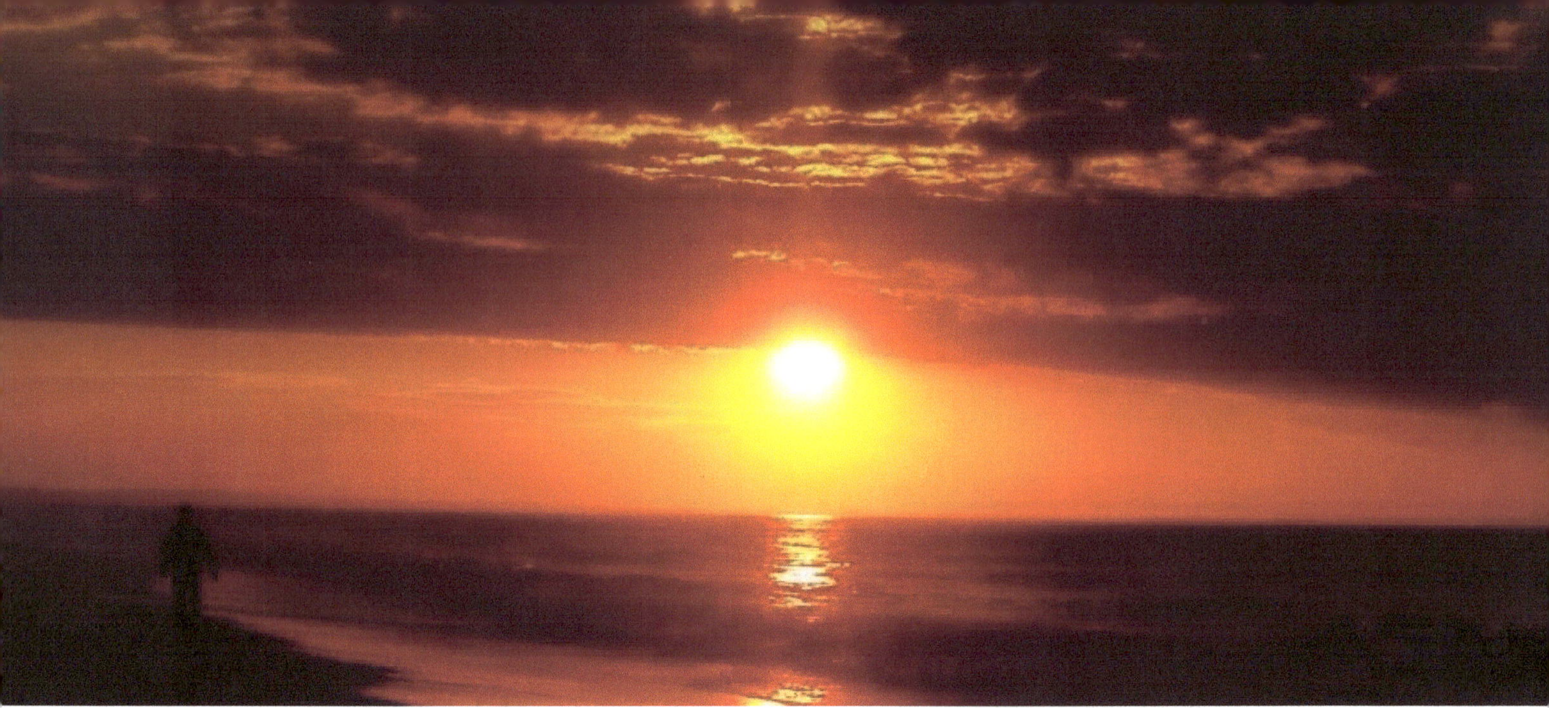

What Might Have Been

By Nicole Bingaman

I am the mother of three amazing sons. Just a few years ago, my husband and I were preparing for our life in an empty nest and all the changes that would bring. In a matter of seconds, the world as we knew it blew up. And we now realize that our nest may never be empty after all.

Our oldest son, Taylor, would be the one who transported our family into the world of traumatic brain injury (TBI). Three-and-a-half years ago, on Thanksgiving Eve, Taylor fell down the stairs in our home. He suffered a severe TBI, and those moments changed us from the second they started. In time they would re-define the very fiber of our family.

> "I have to confess that social media can be a dangerous place for someone who is grieving."

Lately, I have had this recurring image in my mind of what might have been. I have to confess that social media can be a dangerous place for someone who is grieving. The kind of grief doesn't really matter, but as many reading this know, ambiguous loss is often challenging to explain and understand. No matter how often I do it, sharing my truest emotions feels exceptionally difficult.

The night of the fall, Taylor's body and mind were immediately unresponsive and would remain so for several weeks. He finally began his long emergence from a coma while at Bryn Mawr Rehabilitation Hospital outside of Philadelphia. Taylor, with our family by his side, spent many months at Bryn Mawr, while he made both small and large strides. My youngest son referred to that time period as if he were watching his big brother being reborn. The rebirth of Taylor, his emergence, was both glorious and painful to witness, and his recovery continues to impact us in much the same way. There are peaks and valleys, and they often shift from hour to hour. The momentum is not the same as it was in the beginning, but the pendulum between acceptance and grief is always swinging. It never seems to settle for long, forever swaying while the moments that I wish could return, feel like they slip further away.

Now that I am part of the brain injury community, I understand that Taylor, in a sense, is one of the fortunate ones. Taylor can communicate clearly. He is able to execute many parts of his self-care routine. He can eat, walk, talk and exercise. More importantly, he can express love, sadness, happiness, sorrow, joy and all that lies in between those emotions. On the downside, Taylor suffers with a major seizure disorder, numerous cognitive deficits and lacks insight into the reality of his injury. He requires 24-7 supervision, and deals daily with the emotional fallout from an event of this magnitude, as do his brothers and parents.

Recently in the land of sharing which exists via social media circles and on more personal levels, many of my friends' children, who are the same age as Taylor, are announcing their engagements, making huge leaps in their careers, moving out of their childhood home, while continuing to emotionally reside in the nest of safety that the love of family has afforded them. They are spreading their wings, and not only learning to fly, but actually taking off. Some of them are even having babies.

Because I have two other sons in my nest, I know that these times of change and growth are not always easy on a parent's heart, but in truth the greatest wish we have for the little people who were entrusted to us, is that their adulthood leads them to happiness and contentment.

Recently I have been listening to and truly hearing the lyrics of a song that says, "If I had to choose a day that I'd remember, my friend I'd say that would be the one." I clearly remember a day that I will always cherish with Taylor. It is a day that has haunted me since his fall. It is a day that I never want to forget, as much as sometimes the remembering hurts.

That day, I was sitting on the kitchen counter, and the sun was shining in the window behind Taylor. He was getting ready to graduate from high school, and we both had the sense that our lives were about to change. Taylor did not really want to grow up so fast, nor did I want him to. Taylor opened his heart to me that day, and we shared a moment I will forever treasure.

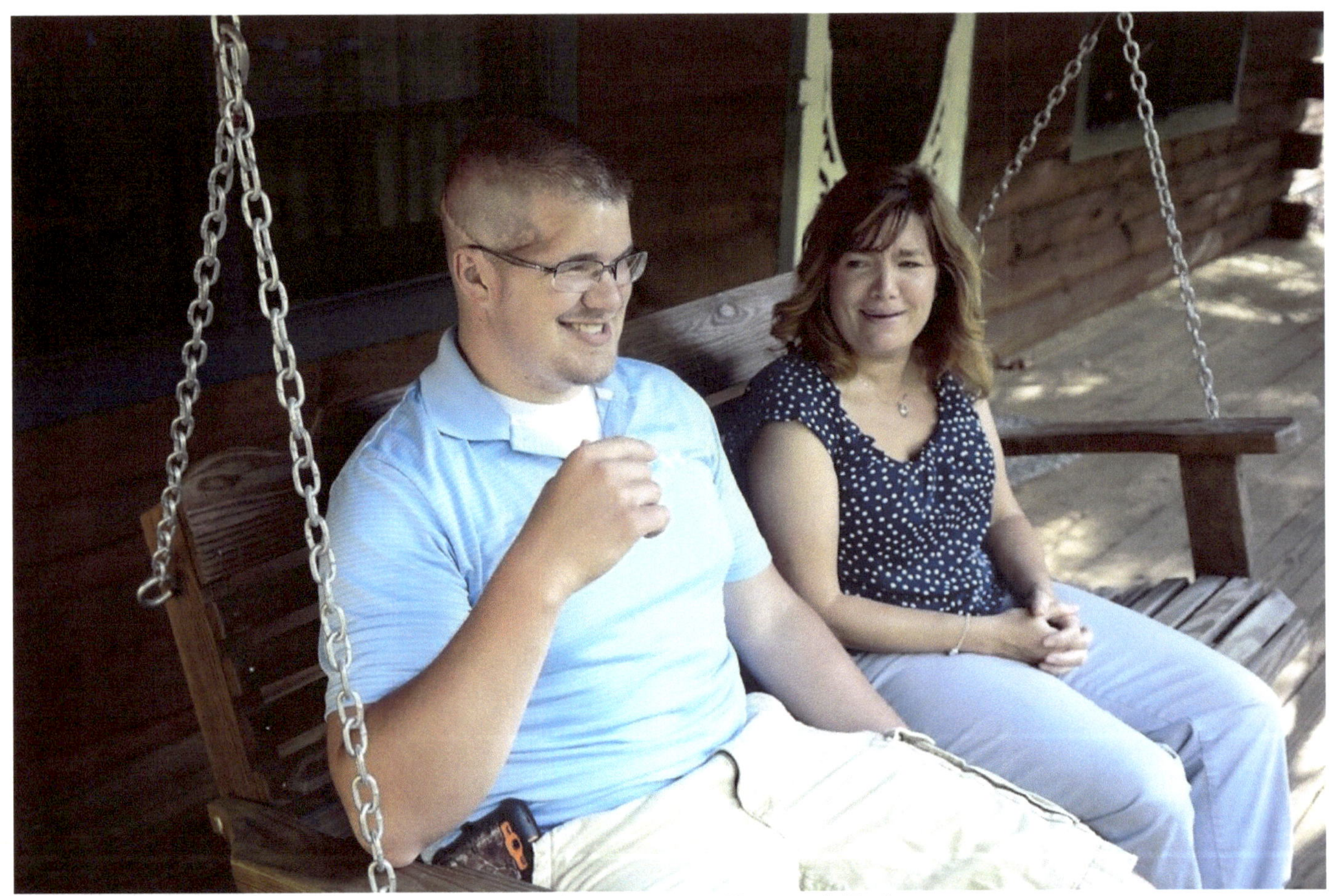

Nicole Bingaman at Home with Taylor

As time moved on, we stepped through many days of change. And Taylor faced them with a confidence and certainty that was admirable. As Taylor's mother it was always magical for me to see him evolving into more of a man than a boy. The one thing that often halted the process in my mind was that Taylor had a baby face. He had the face of a little prince from the moment he was born, and his rosy cheeks and innocence remained a delight to me. I had a small collection of dreams for him, and these were things that I never for a moment thought would not come to be. Now I find myself wondering if there is a box that I should put them in, so that I don't have to face them every day.

Taylor was a man's man. He loved the outdoors, hunting and fishing. He was excited when he bought his first truck with money he had saved for years, and when he got his first "real" job, he saved to buy an even bigger, better and louder truck. He liked to work, and appreciated his skills and energy.

He was known as both a hard and dedicated worker within his HVAC company. Taylor had very few serious romances and was still figuring out that part of life.

In the time before the fall, I wanted more for Taylor. I wanted him to explore more, to branch out a bit, and to see what life might be like discovering a sunset in a new place. Taylor grew up and lived in a small town his entire life, and before he decided to stay there forever, I wanted him to see other parts of the world. He was intelligent, bright and driven, and I pictured him spreading his wings.

Now I realize that those things that Taylor wanted for himself… stability, to own a home, a life-partner and a family were what would make Taylor happy in life. Those dreams that he had appeared to be simple, but they were treasures, and gifts that should not have been taken for granted. To be happy, to be loved, to work and provide for yourself daily, and to share with his loved ones, those things were enough.

For now I am not ready to lay the dreams I held for Taylor to rest. Doing so is just too hard for me, and I don't fully know what the future holds. I find comfort in the improvements he continues to make, and I am grateful every day for the fact that I can still be a witness to his changing, growing and adjusting to this new life. When I see the person that used to be my son, in the reserved part of my memory, I whisper to him…I miss you. All the while working in love, to accept the person he has become.

Meet Nicole Bingaman

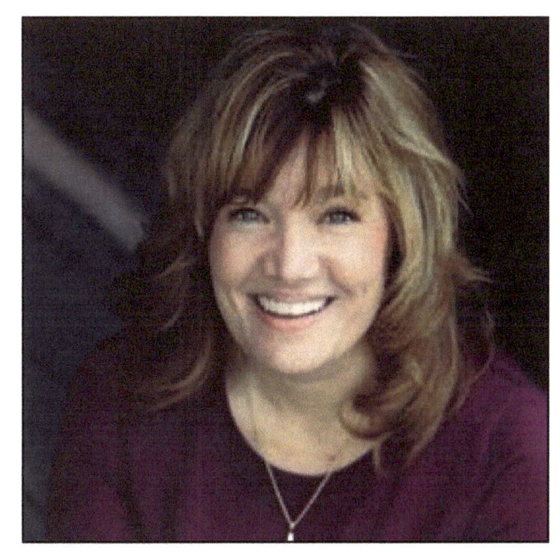

Nicole has worked in the human service field for over twenty years. Since Taylor's injury Nicole has become an advocate and spokesperson within the TBI community, speaking at conferences, trainings and events for professionals and lay people to understand the impact of TBI within a family.

Nicole's book "Falling Away From You" was published and released in 2015. Nicole continues to share Taylor's journey on Facebook. Nicole firmly believes in the mantra "Love Wins."

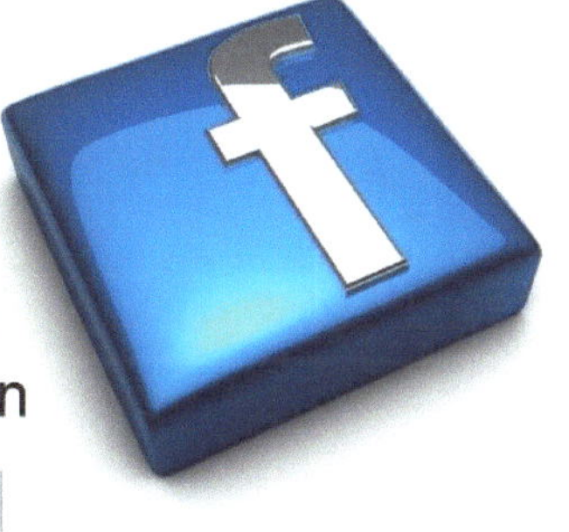

The Many Faces of Traumatic Brain Injury

A Photo Essay

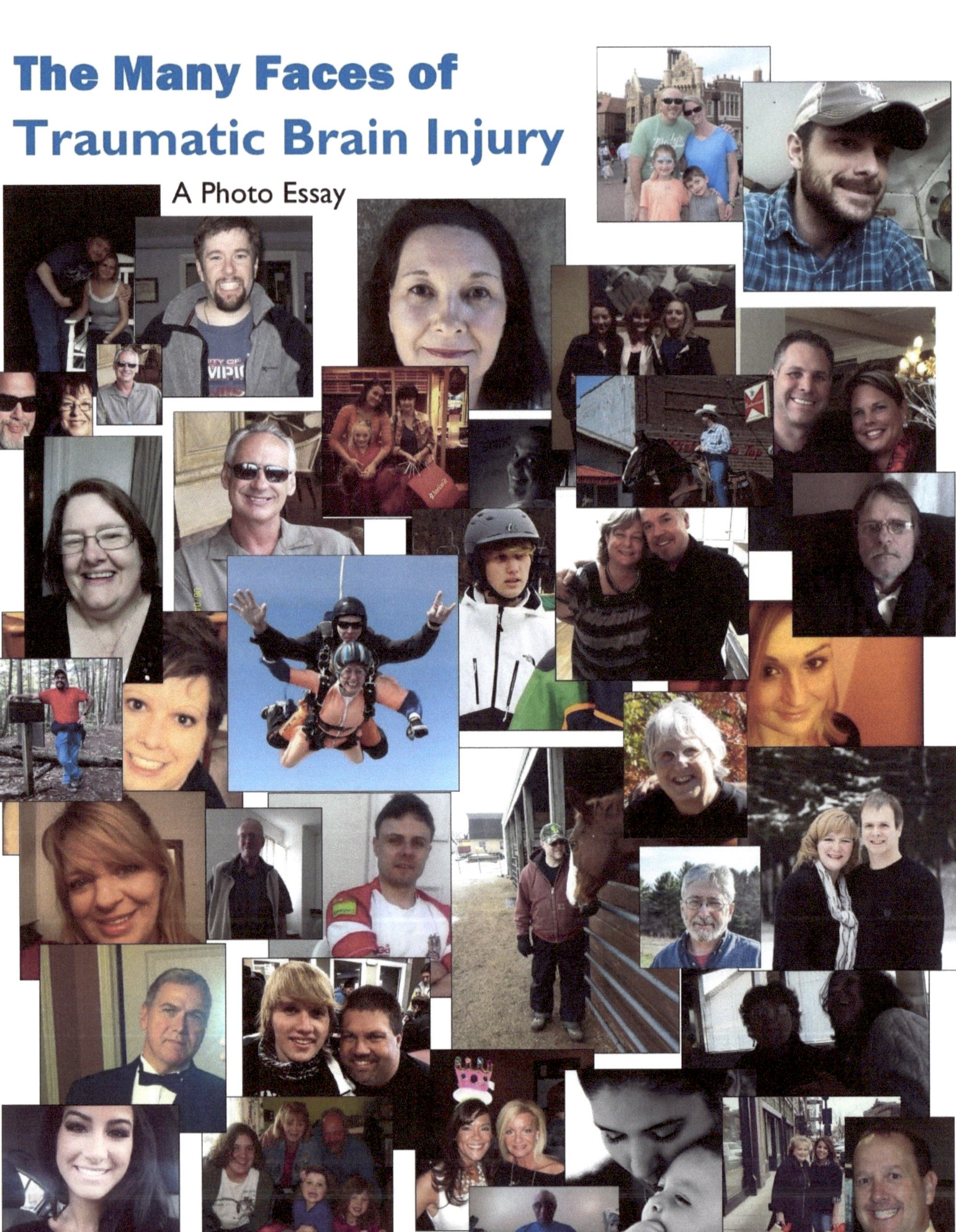

A Caregiver's Journey

By Lydia Greear

On June 29, 2013, at 11:58 pm in Lexington, Kentucky, a speeding vehicle hit my son while he was walking in a crosswalk. He suffered life threatening injuries including a Traumatic Brain Injury. He was rushed within minutes to the local University Medical Center for urgent care. Our son was 37 years old rooming with a friend near the scene of the accident. He was with another friend who witnessed the entire accident.

My husband and I were on a trip to France. We had two more weeks of travel and site seeing. We had been out all day with friends in Paris and our cell phones had no battery power. We arrived at our hotel and put the phones on the charger. Once the charge was renewed to the phones there were text messages, voice messages, and Facebook messages from our two children in the US and others trying to contact us. "Call home, it's urgent," was the theme of every message.

We called them around 11 PM Paris time to learn of the tragic accident. In shock we sat for what seemed hours not knowing what to think or do. Sometime after 1:00 AM local time we contacted the airline to see what options we had to get home as soon as possible.

The airline accommodated us easily and the next day we travelled from the nearest international airport to Lexington, where we rushed to the hospital to see our son. The doctors had taken him to surgery to relieve pressure on the brain and we waited to hear the news. Hours passed and with no information from the medical staff we had to leave to get a hotel room. We left contact information for them to call immediately.

Early the next morning we had still not received any news about our son. We called the hospital and they said he was still in recovery. We rushed to the hospital and found that he had been moved from the original Urgent Care room. After some confusion we were able to finally find our son. A chaplain came to us and was there to prepare us for what we would see.

> "After some confusion we were able to finally find our son. A chaplain came to us and was there to prepare us for what we would see."

Our son was lying in a highly elevated hospital bed with tubes and drains all around him. Several bottles of fluids were above his head. He had a combination of dried blood and blacktop caked in his head. He had an extremely large stitched area from the front part of his head to the back. We were told this was where the neurosurgeon stitched up the injury. He had fresh bandages around the drain tube on the right side of his head.

We waited and prayed. We asked questions. We were still stunned and had no way to know what had happened that night. Our son had no belongings because everything was taken to the "drying" room at the local police station. The young man with our son had recovered a piece of a black guitar he was carrying when the accident occurred.

For nineteen days we waited for him to give signs of life and awaken from his coma. His first gesture was to squeeze the hand of the doctor and lift his thumbs. His eyes opened, and we were not sure what he was seeing. He had a broken leg and his nose had several fractures.

For the next two years he would slowly recover from this TBI. Doctors first told us that this experience takes 18-24 months to know what normal looks like. After twenty-nine months we still don't know what normal looks like.

We accomplished the government medical coverage and even were fortunate to have an "Acquired Brain Injury Waiver" to compensate all other expenses related to his rehabilitation. These waivers are lengthy in process and I was able to acquire the waiver in one week.

Today, our son can walk and talk. He perseverates (repetition of confused words or phrases) vocally and also in behavior. He has a frontal lobe brain injury. We felt it was best to place him in a Community NeuroRestorative facility where he has received Occupational Therapy, Speech Language Pathology, Behavioral Counseling, and Life Skills Therapies.

The challenges are as present today as they were in the first days while he was comatose. We walk in the dark daily on what is best for him.

I press forward with hope. I have personally spent every two weeks since his entry into the NeuroRestorative facility traveling from my home in Florida to Kentucky. He doesn't remember me being there. He knows that I come to see him but has no concept of how often or for how long.

Doctors first told us that this experience takes 18-24 months to know what normal looks like. After twenty-nine months we still don't know what normal looks like.

His physiatrist told us early on that there is no proof he will heal faster if he is at home without therapies or in a facility. The behaviors he exhibits (agitation, frustration, inappropriate yelling and aggression) are still prevalent. His behavior therapist works diligently to help him be more aware of his actions and body language.

It is difficult for him to understand why he is in a facility. He has no compassion or acceptance of so many people working with him every day. Yet, he has never missed a day of therapy in two years.

We do not know what the future holds. I have kept regular records of every aspect of our son's care and my visits with him. He has two children with his ex-wife. All of his friends have moved on with their lives.

In the beginning people were near to us and wanted to stay informed about what was going on with our son. Now we rarely hear from them. His siblings, his children, and his friends don't visit him at all. My husband and I continue to walk this journey on our own.

Meet Lydia Greear

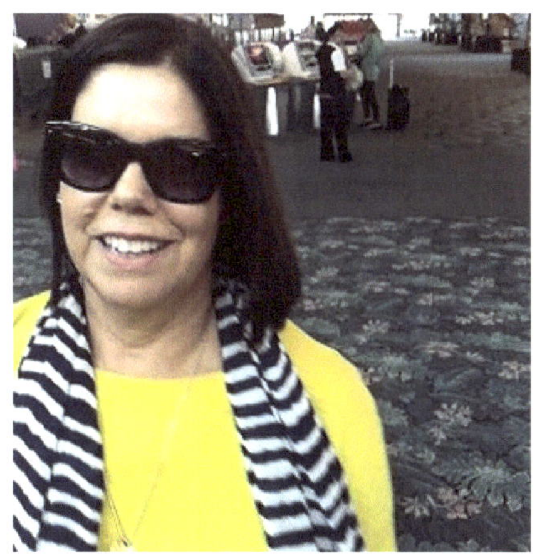

Lydia Greear lives in Florida with her husband of 40 years, Asa. They have three children together, and six grandchildren. She earned a bachelor's degree in sociology from the University of Kentucky. She is a licensed fitness instructor and certified personal trainer, and is also an active member of the Anastasia Baptist Church in St. Augustine. Lydia enjoys traveling, and has spent 14 years living in Paris, France, Benin and Côte d'Ivoire.

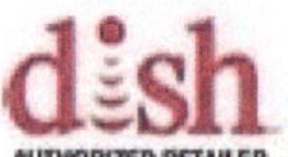

dish
AUTHORIZED RETAILER

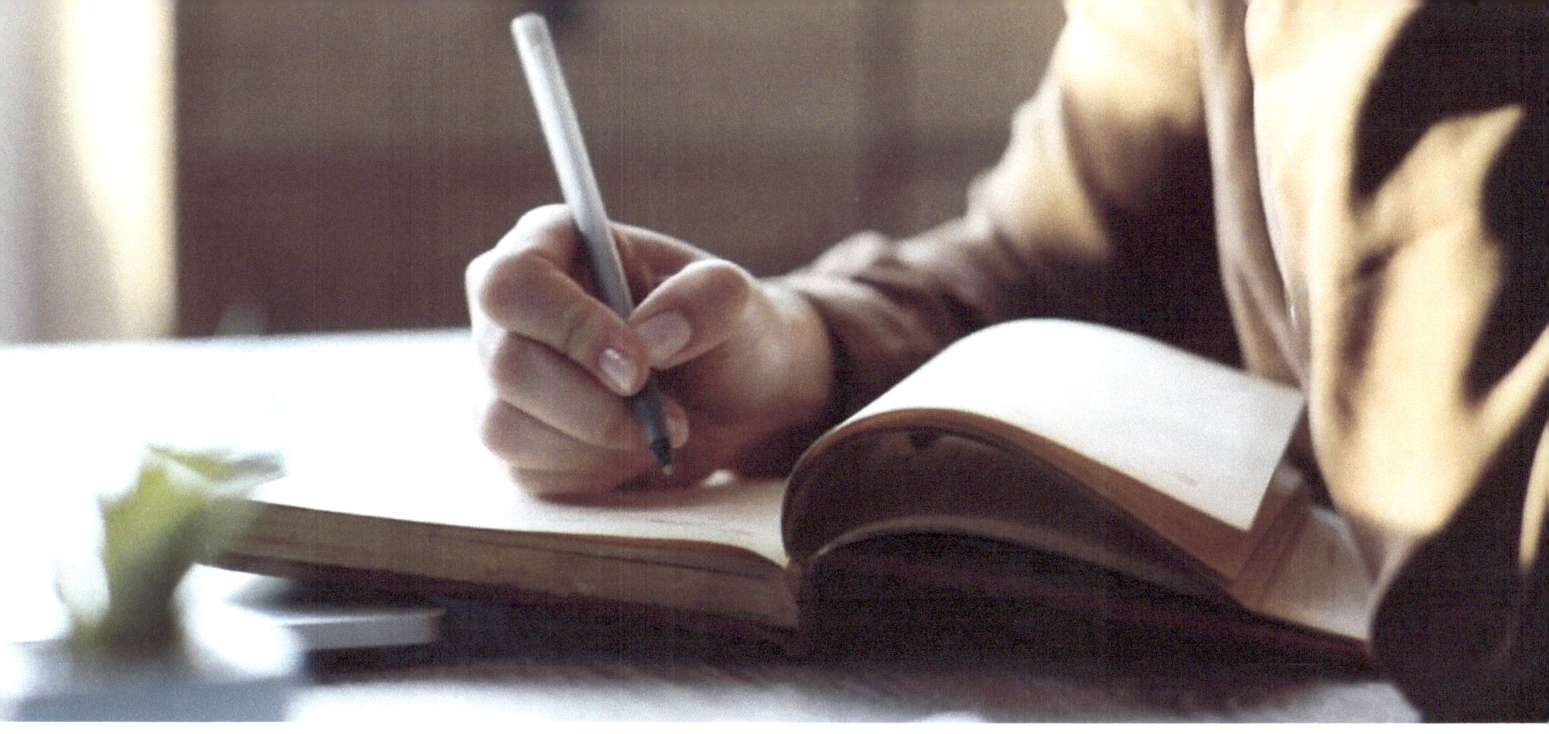

Journaling a New Story

By Barbara Stahura

When a brain injury happens, the familiar story of a life can be altered in ways not possible with any other kind of injury or illness. So much you knew about yourself—the wealth of information you depended upon to lead your life—can blur or disappear, leaving you stranded and struggling in an unknown place. Along with cognitive and emotional challenges, you may face challenges with your physical abilities. You can feel as though you've been kidnapped to an alien planet where nothing is familiar, and you are lost in dangerous territory.

> "Despite being diagnosed with secondary traumatic stress, journaling allowed me to hold on and cope with the overpowering uncertainty, fear, and anxiety."

Family caregivers can feel equally bewildered, as well as terrified. I certainly did when my husband sustained a serious traumatic brain injury more than a decade ago. But my journal offered a safe sanctuary where I could pour out my deepest thoughts and feelings without judgment or criticism. Writing somehow made them more manageable. Despite being diagnosed with secondary traumatic stress, journaling allowed me to hold on and cope with the overpowering uncertainty, fear, and anxiety.

As I've found during eight years of guiding journaling groups for people with brain injury and family caregivers, telling your story through journaling can enhance the healing process. "Healing" here does not mean restoring your injured brain to its former functioning or your life to the way it used to be.

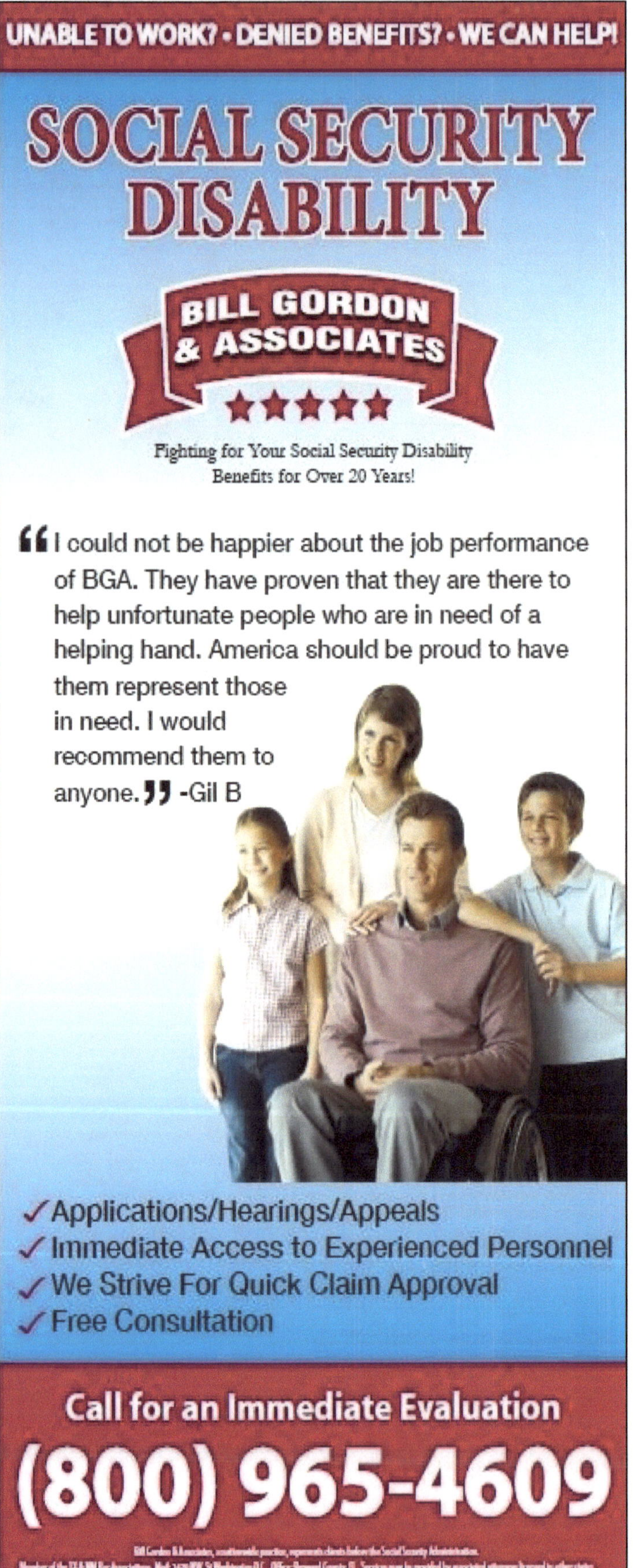

Instead, it means finding healthy ways to become aware of, accept, and acknowledge what has happened so that you can move forward into your new post-injury story. Journaling, for even five or ten minutes at a time on a regular basis, can help release you from yearning for the past and open positive doors to your envisioned future.

How to Journal

There are no rules in journaling, except perhaps to date all your entries. So don't worry about correct spelling, grammar, or punctuation. You need not be a "good" writer. Simply write in whatever way is comfortable for you. You can write on paper or use a keyboard. If a brain injury prohibits you from doing either, you can speak your entries into a recording device, use speech-recognition software, or find a trusted confidante who will scribe your words without judgment or changes.

Keeping your journal private allows you to write honestly. But if you occasionally write an entry that you never want anyone to read, you can tear it out and destroy it. The benefit of journaling comes in the writing, not in preserving what you write.

To begin, you can simply pick up your pen or put your hands on the keyboard. But it's helpful to create a structure for yourself by starting with a prompt (for example: Today I feel… or, The most important thing I can do now…) You can experiment with various techniques such as Dialogue or Unsent Letter, or even setting a time limit.

If you're writing about a traumatic experience, don't simply begin writing with no structure in place. Even something as simple as a five-minute limit can help you avoid writing yourself off an emotional cliff with no way back to safety. Stop writing if you feel yourself getting unusually upset. And over time, try to keep a balance between positive and negative so that you don't end up endlessly ruminating on the darker aspects of your life.

After a brain injury, you might not be able to write much or for very long. Do whatever you can, and please don't judge yourself harshly. As your condition improves, you will be able to write more. If you're a caregiver, you might have difficulty finding time for self-care, but know that you can journal in only five or ten minutes at a time. A small journal will fit in a purse or pocket, and you can write wherever you are.

As you continue journaling, you will have written memories of your healing and of how far you have come since brain injury altered your life. And there, in those words on the page, you—whether survivor or caregiver—have created the foundation on which to build the new story that will carry you into the future.

Meet Barbara Stahura

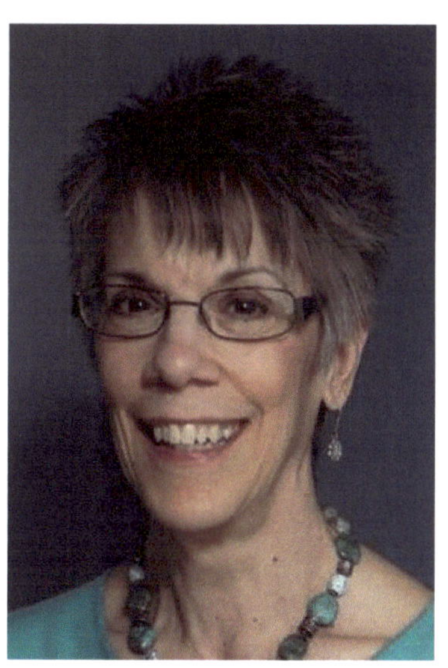

Barbara is a Certified Journal Facilitator and has guided people in harnessing the power of therapeutic journaling for healing and well-being since 2007. She facilitates local journaling groups for people with brain injury and for family caregivers. Co-author of the acclaimed "After Brain Injury: Telling Your Story," the first journaling book for people with brain injury, she lives in Indiana with her husband, a survivor of brain injury.

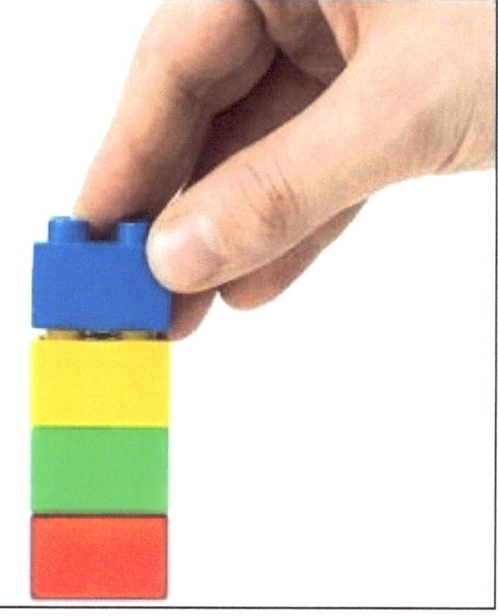

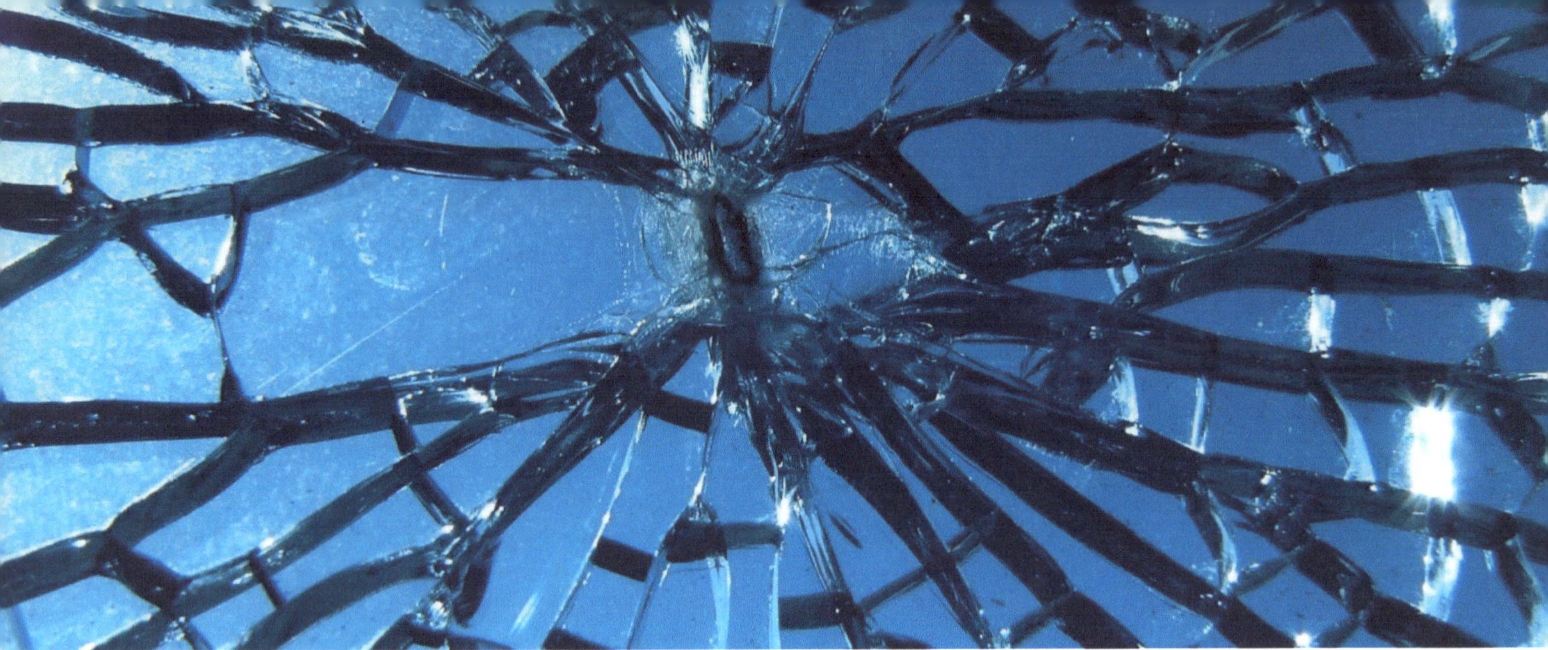

Shattering the One-Year Myth

By David A. Grant

As the years continue to pass by, I have gained one thing that I was not capable of having early on after my injury - I have gained a perspective that comes with time.

Like so many others who share my fate, I get a bit reflective every year around TBI anniversary time. It's a bit of a "take stock" time for me as I look at where I am today – compared to where I was. I now allow myself to look to the future with hope, a realistic hope that I will continue to heal.

But there was a day that someone stole my hope and left me completely and utterly devastated.

I'm a big fan of taking personal inventory. A year after I was struck down by a teenaged driver while I was cycling, I decided it was time. I had heard a lot about neuropsychological testing. It was time to see how many of my marbles remained. I wanted a clearer understanding of my deficits so that I could have a starting point, a place to begin the next chapter of my healing.

> "As we reviewed the results of my testing it was clear that my assessment was not quite what we expected."

After hours of grueling testing that took place over the course of several days, I sat down with my wife, Sarah, and the neuropsychologist. As we reviewed the results of my testing it was clear that my assessment was not quite what we expected.

"David, you are in the bottom five percentile in the areas of complex problem solving and verbal recall," he said as dryly as if giving driving directions to a stranger. This fact alone was shocking enough. But there were more sucker punches to my soul awaiting.

"You are permanently disabled, and any gains you have from here on out will be small at best," he shared, as my wife and I sat there trying to comprehend the gravity of his diagnosis.

Still keeping a stiff upper lip, I asked about scheduling a neuropsychological test a year out, suggesting that we could use this first test as a benchmark to measure future gains.

"There is no need, your gains will be insignificant at best," came the authoritative answer. As our visit wound down, there was a final hope-stealing shot across my bow.

"Most brain injury survivors see an IQ drop after their injuries. It's clear that you were a very intelligent man before your accident. Even losing some of your IQ, you should be able to get by relatively okay now," he propounded, as we were getting ready to leave his office.

Many years have passed since that meeting. Swimming in a sea with other survivors over the years, I have heard this same misinformation shared over and over again – after a year, you are as good as you are going to get. Please check your HOPE at the door. No need for optimism. Go directly to TBI jail, do not pass Go, do not collect $200. Hunker down and just grin and bear it. You are lucky enough just to be alive.

Balderdash!

As time continues to pass, I now recognize this kind of advice for what it is: old-school science. The old-school TBI science was simple and easy.

You are permanently disabled, and any gains you have from here on out will be small at best.

After a year, any gains would be small. Thankfully, a new school of science is now dominating the national brain injury narrative. New school science embraces neuroplasticity and challenges the archaic belief that recovery has an end game. New school science embraces the hidden power of the brain and human body. New school science says that as long as you have a heartbeat, you will continue to heal. And best of all, new school science is a science of hope - hope that the way things are today are not how they will be next year, or in five years.

One of the first to push old school science to the side was Dr. Jill Bolte-Taylor. In her book, My Stroke of Insight, she speaks of measurable gains through the eight-year mark. Last year at this time, I attended a conference in Maine. The keynote presenter, who is also a doctor and the parent of a survivor, took to the podium in front of her peers and continued this new narrative.

 "As a medical community, we got it wrong when we told you that recovery was over in a year. We got it wrong," she shared. You could have heard a pin drop.

I hold no ill will, anger or resentment to the well-intentioned doctor who temporarily stole my hope. He was only preaching what his old-school science had taught him. As the tide continues to turn, more and more members of the medical and professional community are letting go of the one-year myth. The Dark Ages of brain injury recovery are slowly fading into the past. I need only look at my own life to see some of the long-term gains.

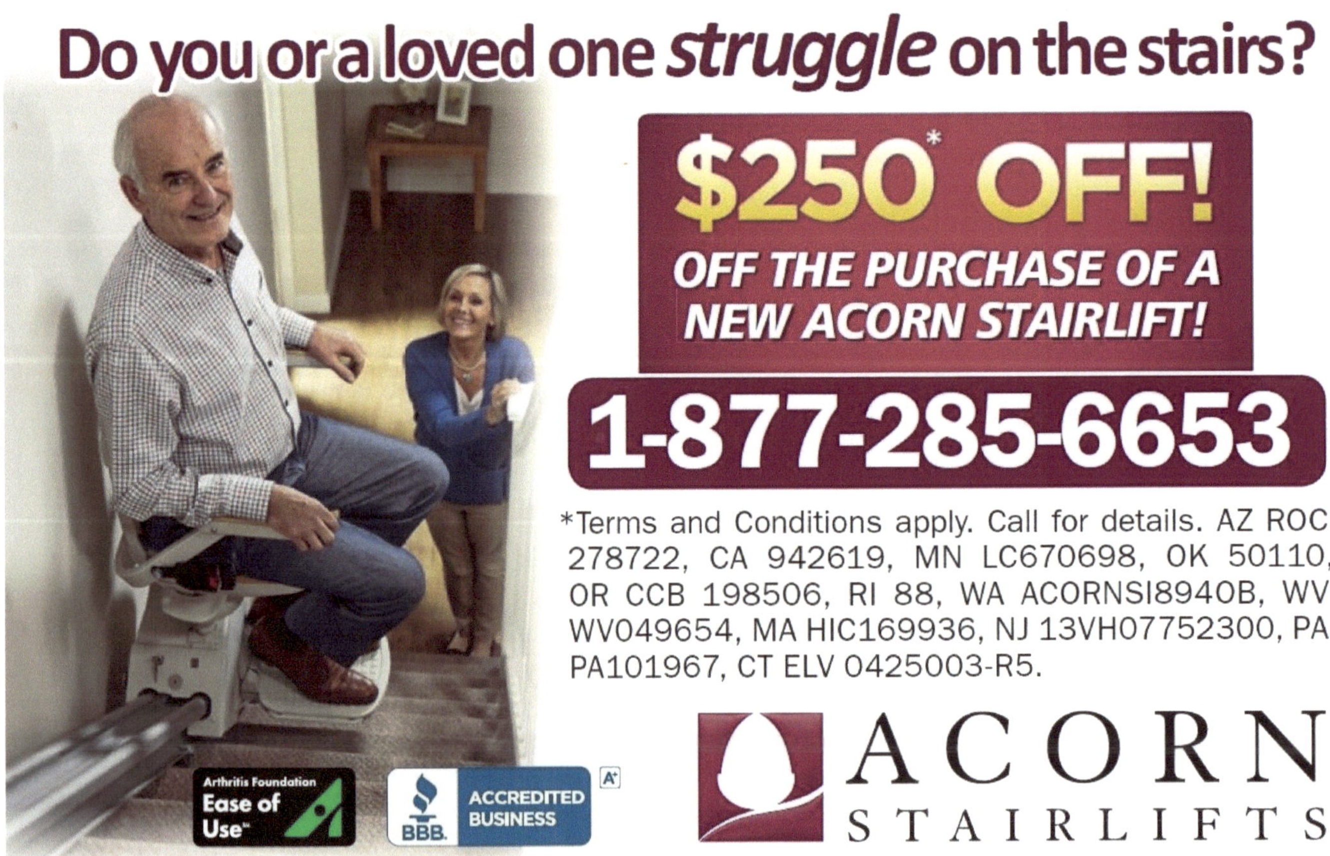

At two years out, my vertigo almost ceased. At three years out, I was again able to work beyond 2:00 PM every day. At four years out, I was able to read books again – something I thought I had lost forever. The list goes on.

Today I have real hope – hope that I will continue my path toward recovery. Not "whistling in the dark" hope, this is true hope based on my life experience as well as emerging science. I don't kid myself for a moment because I know I'll never be who I was.

But today, where I am going is so much more important than where I was.

Meet David A. Grant

David A. Grant is a traumatic brain injury survivor from Salem, NH. In addition to publishing HOPE Magazine, David is also a staff writer for Brainline.org as well as a contributing writer to Chicken Soup for the Soul, Surviving Traumatic Brain Injuries. David is a board member of the Brain Injury Association of New Hampshire. When he's not working, David can be found cycling the back roads of southern New Hampshire.

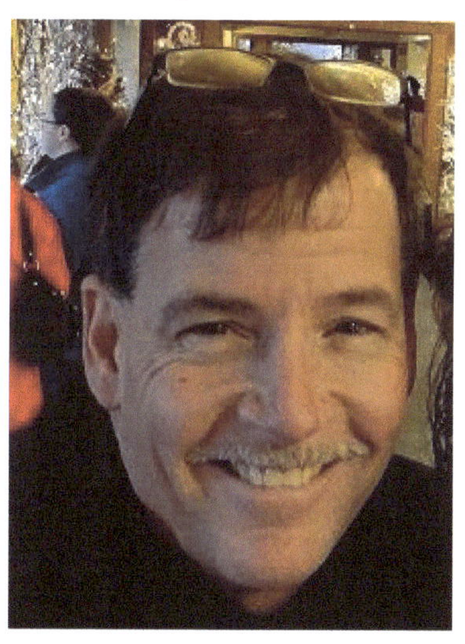

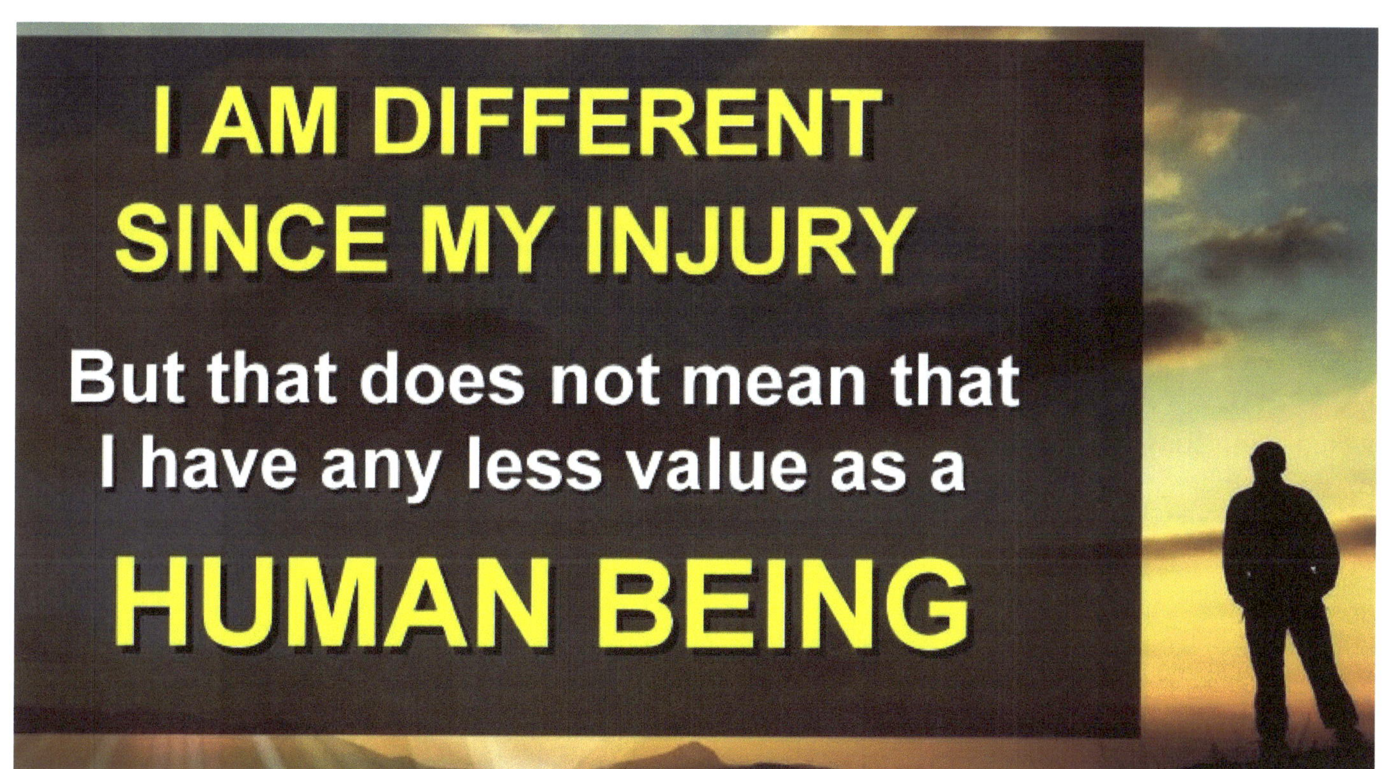

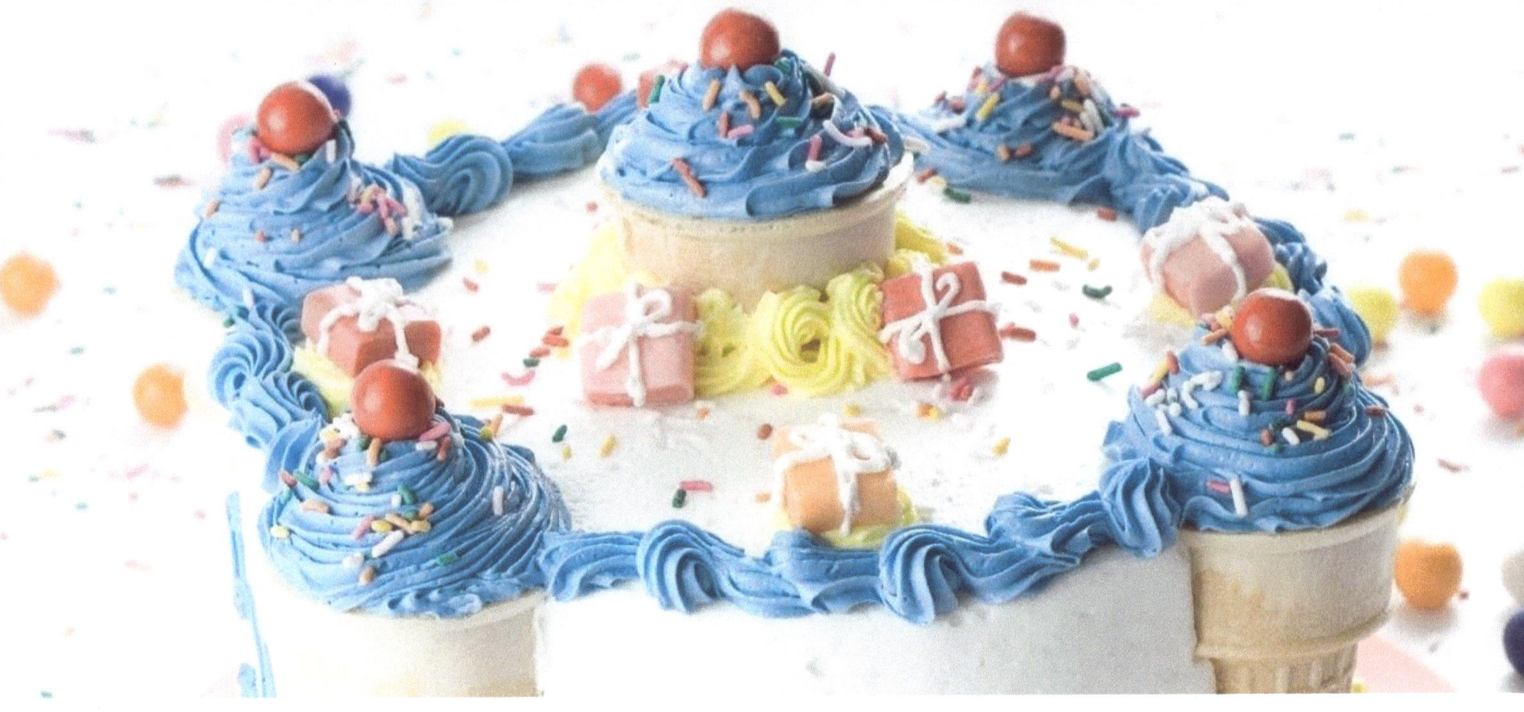

Anniversaries

By Carole Starr

The brain injury that changed my life forever occurred on July 6th, 1999. One challenge in accepting my new life was coping with the anniversary date of my accident. I used to think about the car accident on the 6th of every month. That thinking faded on its own within the first year. However, for many years, every July 6th I would remember and grieve more acutely my life that was. I would more intensely miss the woman who was able to manage and excel at many activities.

During this time, my view of my former self and her past would become rosier, colored by the sense of loss I felt. My ongoing brain injury symptoms and limitations would frustrate me more. I would get angry at myself because I hadn't progressed further and in the process, I would completely discount all the gains I'd made. I needed a strategy to cope with the feelings of sadness and loss brought on by my brain injury anniversary date.

> "I needed a strategy to cope with the feelings of sadness and loss brought on by my brain injury anniversary date."

It took me eight anniversaries and the help of family and friends to come up with a strategy that worked for July 6th. It's one that I use every year now. This strategy has transformed anniversary time from a day of intense sadness to a day of reflection and even celebration. I now view my anniversary day as my second birthday and commemorate it as such.

I'm sharing my strategy in the hopes that it helps others. The anniversary strategy involves four important components.

* Do not be alone
* Remember and celebrate your progress
* Plan life-affirming activities
* Try something new

Do not be alone. It's never a good idea to be all alone on such a meaningful day. It's too easy to allow yourself to brood about what was your life. Instead, spend time with an upbeat person or persons who can show you kindness and compassion.

Remember and celebrate your progress. It's easy to forget just how much progress you've made since your brain injury, especially around anniversary time. You may think that your accomplishments now are insignificant next to your pre-injury ones. However, when compared to the early days of your recovery, I'm sure the progress is downright stunning.

And that progress, however small and however slow, will continue. As you progress, it's not fair to judge your new life by the standards of your old one. That kind of judgment will only make anniversary time more painful. If instead you compare apples to apples - start of your new life with a brain injury to your present stage of recovery - anniversary time becomes less a time to mourn and more a time to celebrate just how far you've come.

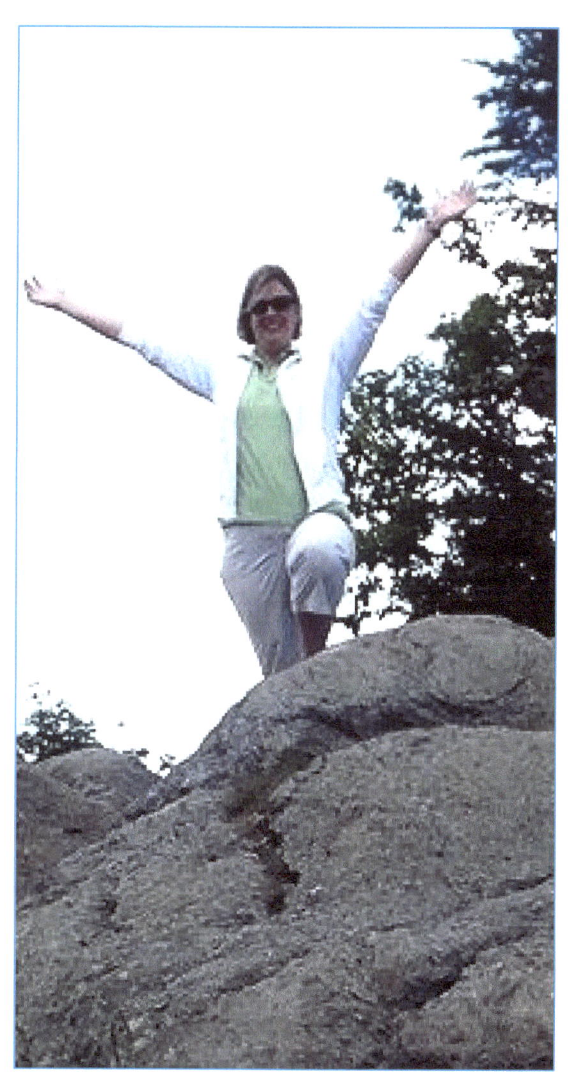

Plan Life-Affirming Activities. It's important to think about how you'd like to spend your anniversary day. Planning and doing something fun and fulfilling serves two purposes. The planning process itself can distract you during the days or weeks before the actual anniversary and give you something to look forward to. A life-affirming activity on the day itself will prevent you from thinking too much about your pre-injury life. Whatever activity you choose, it should fill your soul and respect your current abilities.

The last thing you want is to choose something too difficult that will only frustrate and depress you. Depending on your abilities, you may plan one activity or several. You may require help planning or you may be able to do it on your own. Perhaps you'd like to spend time with several people or maybe just one. You may even choose to pursue a solo activity. Just be sure not to spend all day alone, even if all you can do is talk to someone on the phone. Regarding the type of activity, there is no right or wrong choice. It should be life-affirming to you. Some possibilities are spending time with family and friends, doing a craft/art project, volunteering, gardening, reading to a child, listening to/playing music, spending time in nature, cooking a special meal, building something, playing with a pet, exercising, or whatever else you can dream up. Listen to your inner voice for guidance and just have fun!

Try something new. This is my favorite part of the anniversary day strategy. Do something you've never done before. Since you got a new life with your brain injury, anniversary day should be commemorated by trying something new. The life affirming activity and the new activity may be one in the same, but they don't have to be. The activity doesn't need to be long or complicated, just new. For example, the first year I implemented this strategy, I simply went with friends to a restaurant and ordered a dish I'd never eaten before.

Over the years, my new activities have gotten bigger as my capabilities have expanded. It's most important to try something that's in line with whatever your current abilities are. So unless you're truly, truly up for it, I wouldn't recommend anything too exotic, like bungee jumping off the tallest building you can find! What the activity represents is far more important than the activity itself.

As with any life-affirming strategy, planning and doing something new can serve as a distraction and give you something to look forward to.

Over the years, July 6th has been a day when I've gone to the botanical gardens with my best friend, created collages with my brain injury support group, watched a rubber duck race, ridden a gondola up a mountain, hiked to a waterfall with my family, taken pictures at the beach and eaten many more new foods.

I never would have dreamed it early on, but I can honestly say I now enjoy July 6th. Yes, I will always know that it's the day brain injury changed my life forever, but with the help of my strategy, it's been transformed into a positive, celebratory, forward-looking day. I hope this anniversary strategy can help you do the same.

Meet Carole Starr

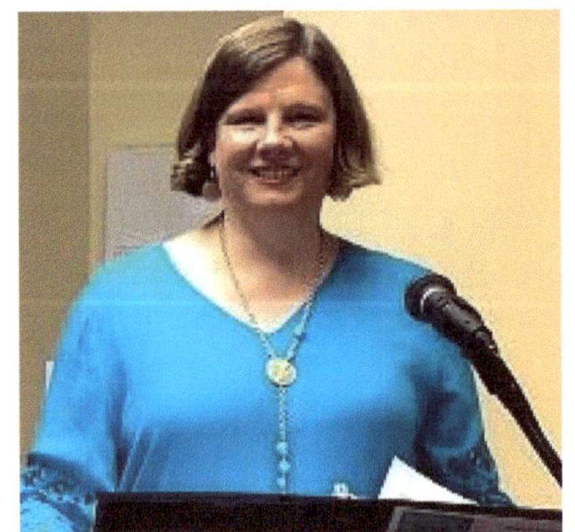

Carole is a brain injury keynote speaker, the Founder and Facilitator of Brain Injury Voices and the creator of the traveling photography exhibit Resilience: Moving Forward after Adversity. She can be contacted through the Brain Injury Voices website at www.braininjuryvoices.org.

News & Views

We hope that you have enjoyed this month's issue of HOPE Magazine. Over the years, it has been an honor to share the stories of hundreds of survivors with our readers worldwide.

From the inception of our publication, we made a decision to share the reality of brain injury as it is – often difficult and always life-changing.

To attempt to gloss over the reality of the way life really is after brain injury would be to disserve our community.

This month, we featured some of the stories that readers have shared were very helpful. But it doesn't stop there. We are always looking forward, asking the same question: *"How can we best serve the brain injury community?"*

In an upcoming issue, we are going to focus on solutions – things that have helped others as they navigate this new and uncertain road. In our case, support groups have become a mainstay of ongoing recovery.

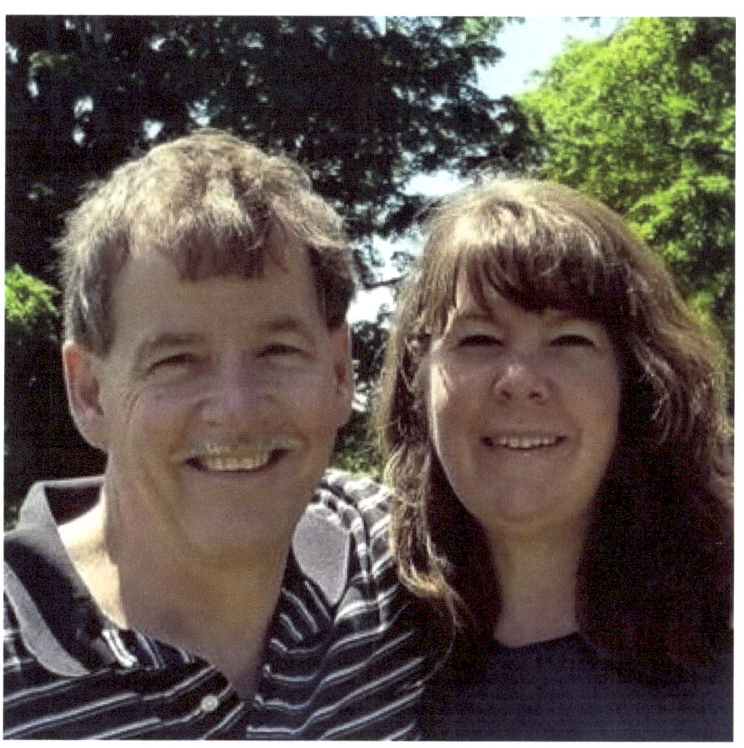

That being said, we are looking for contributors for our upcoming Brain Injury Solutions issue. If you have something that has worked well for you, please consider sharing it with our readers.

You can reach me directly at david@tbihopeandinspiration.com. We strongly encourage you to share your story. You have the ability to help others!

Peace,

David and Sarah